I0703077

Blood Sugar Solution Recipes

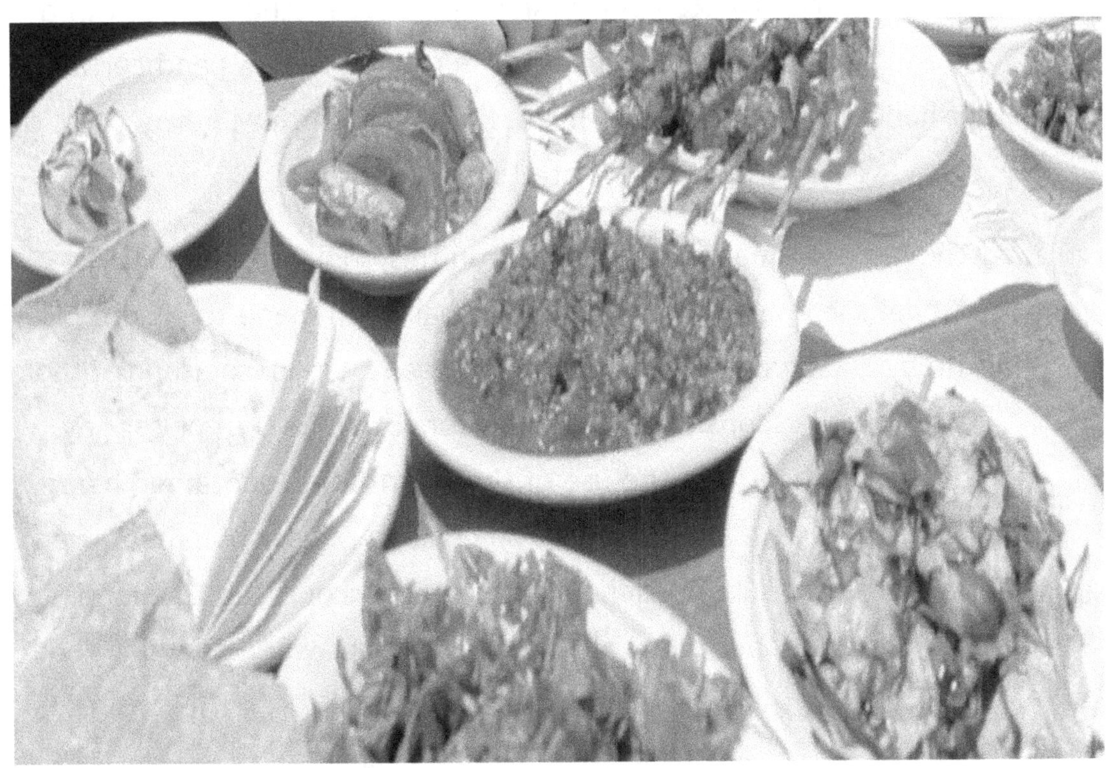

60 Delicious and Easy Recipes to Balance Blood Sugar Naturally

Trends Kitchen

Copyright Page

Copyright © 2024 by Trends Kitchen

All rights reserved. No part of this book may be reproduced, distributed, or transmitted in any form or by any means, including photocopying, recording, or other electronic or mechanical methods, without the prior written permission of Trends Kitchen, except in the case of brief quotations embodied in critical reviews and certain other noncommercial uses permitted by copyright law. For permission requests, write to the publisher.

The recipes, images, and content in this book are intended for personal use only. While every effort has been made to ensure the accuracy and completeness of the recipes, the publisher and author assume no responsibility for any errors or omissions, or for any outcome resulting from the use of the information contained herein. Individual results may vary based on cooking skills, equipment used, and ingredient substitutions. Readers are encouraged to exercise good judgment and follow all safety guidelines when handling food and kitchen equipment.

Table of Contents

Introduction

A few years ago, a close friend of mine, Theresa, had a health scare. She always felt tired, often got dizzy, and had trouble concentrating. After a visit to her doctor, she learned that her blood sugar levels were off the charts. She didn't have diabetes, but her doctor warned that she was dangerously close to prediabetes. This news was a wake-up call for Theresa, and it made me realize how crucial it is to understand and manage blood sugar levels through diet and lifestyle.

What is Blood Sugar?

Blood sugar, or blood glucose, is the amount of sugar present in your blood at any given time. Your body gets glucose from the food you eat, primarily from carbohydrates. These carbohydrates are broken down into glucose, which enters your bloodstream and serves as a vital energy source for your body's cells. Insulin, a hormone produced by the pancreas, helps transport glucose from your blood into your cells to be used for energy.

Maintaining balanced blood sugar levels is very important for overall health. When blood sugar levels are too high or too low, it may lead to serious health problems, including diabetes and hypoglycemia.

The Impact of High and Low Blood Sugar Levels

When blood sugar levels remain high over an extended period, it may lead to hyperglycemia, a condition commonly associated with diabetes. High blood sugar levels can damage blood vessels, nerves, and organs. Symptoms of hyperglycemia include frequent urination, increased thirst, and blurred vision. Over time, chronic high blood sugar may lead to severe complications like heart disease, kidney damage, and vision problems.

Conversely, low blood sugar levels, or hypoglycemia, can be just as dangerous. Hypoglycemia occurs when there isn't enough glucose in your bloodstream to fuel your body's activities. Symptoms include shakiness, sweating, confusion, and in severe cases, loss of consciousness. For people with diabetes, hypoglycemia may result from taking too much insulin or other diabetes medications.

How Diet Affects Blood Sugar

One of the most powerful tools you have to manage your blood sugar levels is your diet. The foods you eat play a significant role in how your body regulates blood sugar. Carbohydrates, proteins, and fats all influence blood sugar differently. Carbohydrates have the most immediate effect on blood sugar levels. When you eat carbs, your body breaks them down into glucose, which causes your blood sugar levels to rise. However, not all carbohydrates are created equal. Simple carbs, found in sugary snacks and white bread, may cause rapid spikes in blood sugar. In contrast, complex carbs, like those in whole grains and vegetables, are broken down more slowly. This leads to a gradual rise in blood sugar.

Proteins and fats have a more moderate effect on blood sugar. Including them in your meals will help slow down the absorption of glucose from carbohydrates. This will lead to a more stable blood sugar response. For instance, pairing a piece of fruit (carb) with a handful of nuts (protein and fat) can prevent a quick spike in blood sugar.

Fiber, a type of carbohydrate that the body can't digest, also plays a crucial role in blood sugar management. Foods high in fiber, such as beans, whole grains, and vegetables, help slow the absorption of sugar, leading to a more gradual increase in blood sugar levels. It's also important to pay attention to the glycemic index (GI) of foods, which measures how quickly a food causes blood sugar levels to rise. Foods with a high GI, like white bread and sugary cereals, cause rapid spikes in blood sugar, while low GI foods, like most fruits, vegetables, and whole grains, lead to slower, more controlled increases.

Key Nutrients for Blood Sugar Control

Managing blood sugar effectively involves focusing on certain key nutrients. These nutrients help regulate insulin and keep blood glucose levels stable.

i.   **Fiber**: Fiber slows down the absorption of sugar, helping to maintain steady blood sugar levels. Foods rich in fiber include vegetables, fruits, legumes, and whole grains.

ii.   **Protein**: Protein helps stabilize blood sugar levels by slowing the digestion and absorption of carbohydrates. Good sources include lean meats, fish, eggs, beans, and nuts.

iii.   **Healthy Fats**: Healthy fats from sources like avocados, nuts, seeds, and olive oil can improve insulin sensitivity and help keep blood sugar levels in check.

iv.   **Magnesium**: Magnesium plays a role in insulin secretion and sensitivity. Foods high in magnesium include leafy greens, nuts, seeds, and whole grains.

    v.   **Chromium**: This mineral enhances the action of insulin. It's found in broccoli, barley, oats, and tomatoes.

Foods to Include

To keep blood sugar levels balanced, it's important to incorporate the right foods into your diet.

Here's a list of foods that will help:

    i.   **Leafy Greens**: Spinach, kale, and other leafy greens are low in calories and carbohydrates but high in fiber and magnesium.

    ii.   **Berries**: Blueberries, strawberries, and raspberries are lower in sugar compared to other fruits and packed with fiber and antioxidants.

    iii.   **Nuts and Seeds**: Almonds, walnuts, chia seeds, and flaxseeds provide healthy fats, protein, and fiber.

    iv.   **Whole Grains**: Oats, quinoa, brown rice, and whole wheat products contain fiber and nutrients that help regulate blood sugar.

    v.   **Legumes**: Beans, lentils, and chickpeas are rich in protein, fiber, and complex carbohydrates that are slowly digested.

    vi.   **Lean Proteins**: Chicken, turkey, fish, and tofu provide essential protein without excess saturated fat.

    vii.   **Non-Starchy Vegetables**: Broccoli, cauliflower, zucchini, and bell peppers are low in carbohydrates and high in fiber.

viii. **Healthy Fats**: Avocados, olive oil, and fatty fish like salmon provide monounsaturated and polyunsaturated fats that help improve insulin sensitivity.

Foods to Avoid

Certain foods can cause blood sugar levels to spike and should be limited or avoided:

i. **Sugary Drinks**: Soda, sweetened coffee, and fruit juices can cause rapid spikes in blood sugar levels.

ii. **Refined Carbohydrates**: White bread, pastries, and pasta made from white flour are quickly broken down into sugar in the bloodstream.

iii. **Sugary Snacks**: Candy, cookies, and cakes are high in added sugars and can lead to blood sugar spikes.

iv. **Processed Foods**: Many processed foods contain high levels of sugar, unhealthy fats, and refined carbohydrates.

v. **High-Glycemic Fruits**: Fruits like bananas, pineapples, and watermelons can cause a quicker rise in blood sugar levels.

vi. **Trans Fats**: Found in many fried and commercially baked products, trans fats can contribute to insulin resistance.

vii. **Alcohol**: Alcohol can cause blood sugar levels to fluctuate and may interfere with diabetes medications.

viii. **High-Fat Dairy**: Full-fat dairy products can increase inflammation and insulin resistance.

Avoiding these foods will certainly help keep your blood sugar levels in check and reduce the risk of complications associated with high blood sugar.

Practical Tips for a Blood Sugar-Friendly Diet

i. **Plan Your Meals:** Planning your meals ahead of time ensures you have the right ingredients on hand and helps prevent last-minute unhealthy choices.

ii. **Portion Control:** Eating smaller, balanced meals throughout the day can help maintain steady blood sugar levels.

iii. **Read Labels:** Pay attention to nutrition labels to avoid hidden sugars and unhealthy fats in processed foods.

iv. **Stay Hydrated:** Drink plenty of water to help your body manage blood sugar levels effectively.

v. **Exercise Regularly:** Physical activity will help your body use insulin more efficiently and lower blood sugar levels.

Understanding and controlling blood sugar is not just about avoiding certain foods—it's about making informed choices that support your body's natural ability to maintain balance. With the right knowledge and tools, you can enjoy a varied and satisfying diet while keeping your blood sugar levels in check. So, on behalf of Trends Kitchen, I'll share in this recipe book, practical and tasty recipes designed to help you manage your blood sugar levels effectively. These recipes focus on low GI ingredients, high fiber content, and balanced macronutrients to ensure steady blood sugar levels throughout the day.

Whether you're looking to prevent blood sugar spikes, manage diabetes, or simply lead a healthier lifestyle, the recipes in this book will be your guide to eating well and feeling great. You'll be taking a significant step towards better health and well-being by incorporating these delicious and easy recipes into your daily routine.

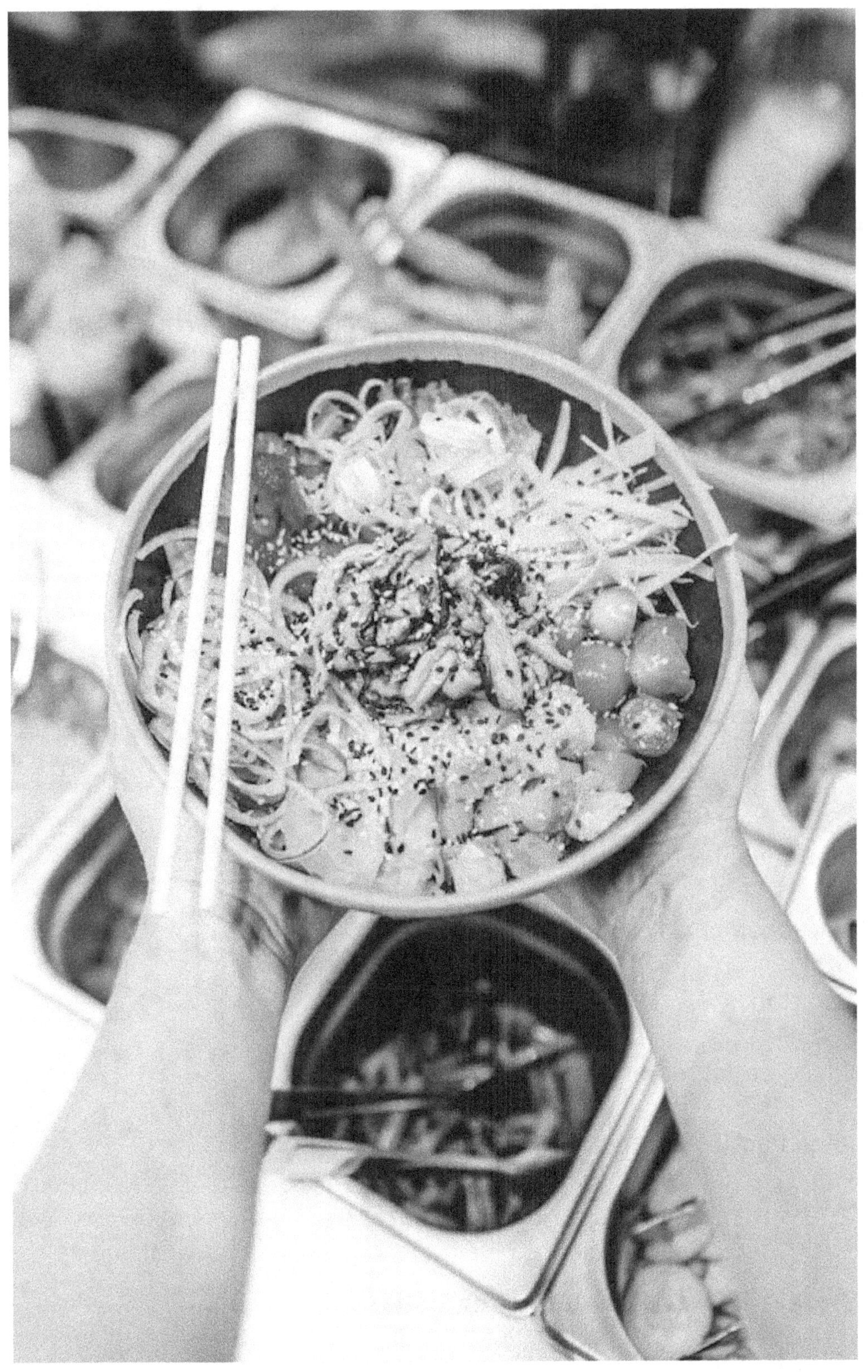

Chapter 1

Breakfast Recipes

• Energizing Morning Smoothies

1. Green Berry Blast

Ingredients:

1 cup fresh spinach

1/2 cup frozen blueberries

1/2 cup frozen strawberries

1 banana

1 cup unsweetened almond milk

1 tablespoon chia seeds

Instructions:

1. Place all ingredients in a blender.

2. Blend until smooth and creamy.

3. Pour into a glass and enjoy immediately.

2. Protein-Packed Peanut Butter Shake

Ingredients:

1 banana

2 tablespoons natural peanut butter

1 scoop vanilla protein powder

1 cup unsweetened almond milk

1 tablespoon ground flaxseed

Instructions:

i.   Add all ingredients to a blender.

ii.   Blend until smooth.

iii.   Serve right away for a quick and filling breakfast.

3. Tropical Mango Delight

Ingredients:

1 cup frozen mango chunks

1/2 cup frozen pineapple chunks

1/2 banana

1 cup coconut water

1/2 cup plain Greek yogurt

Instructions:

1. Combine all ingredients in a blender.

2. Blend until you achieve a smooth consistency.

3. Pour into a glass and savor the tropical flavors.

4. Berry Protein Boost

Ingredients:

1/2 cup frozen mixed berries (blueberries, raspberries, strawberries)

1 scoop whey protein powder

1/2 cup unsweetened almond milk

1/2 cup water

1 tablespoon chia seeds

Instructions:

1. Place all ingredients in a blender.

2. Blend thoroughly until the mixture is smooth.

3. Drink immediately to benefit from the protein and antioxidants.

5. Green Detox Smoothie

Ingredients:

1 cup kale or spinach

1/2 cucumber, sliced

1 green apple, cored and chopped

1 tablespoon fresh lemon juice

1 cup water or coconut water

1 tablespoon chia seeds

Instructions:

1. Put all ingredients into a blender.

2. Blend until smooth and well combined.

3. Enjoy this refreshing detox smoothie right away.

● **Nutritious Breakfast Bowls**

6. Quinoa and Fruit Bowl

Ingredients:

1 cup cooked quinoa

1/2 cup fresh blueberries

1/2 cup fresh strawberries, sliced

1/4 cup almonds, chopped

1 tablespoon chia seeds

1 tablespoon honey (optional)

1/2 cup unsweetened almond milk

Instructions:

1. In a bowl, combine cooked quinoa, blueberries, and strawberries.

2. Sprinkle chopped almonds and chia seeds on top.

3. Drizzle with honey if you prefer a bit of sweetness.

4. Pour almond milk over the mixture.

5. Stir gently and enjoy a nutritious breakfast that helps balance blood sugar levels.

7. Greek Yogurt Parfait with Nuts

Ingredients:

1 cup plain Greek yogurt

1/2 cup granola (low sugar)

1/4 cup walnuts, chopped

1/4 cup sliced almonds

1/2 cup mixed berries (blueberries, raspberries, strawberries)

1 tablespoon flaxseeds

1 tablespoon honey (optional)

Instructions:

1. In a glass or bowl, layer 1/2 cup Greek yogurt.

2. Add a layer of granola, followed by a layer of mixed berries.

3. Sprinkle walnuts, almonds, and flaxseeds over the berries.

4. Repeat the layers, finishing with a drizzle of honey if desired.

5. This parfait is a delicious way to start your day while keeping your blood sugar in check.

8. Oatmeal with Berries and Nuts

Ingredients:

1 cup rolled oats

2 cups water or unsweetened almond milk

1/2 cup mixed berries (blueberries, raspberries, strawberries)

1/4 cup chopped walnuts

1 tablespoon chia seeds

1 tablespoon honey or maple syrup (optional)

1/2 teaspoon cinnamon

Instructions:

1. Cook the oats in water or almond milk according to package instructions.

2. Once cooked, stir in the cinnamon and let it sit for a minute.

3. Top with mixed berries, chopped walnuts, and chia seeds.

4. Drizzle honey or maple syrup on top if desired.

5. Serve warm for a hearty and blood sugar-friendly breakfast.

9. Chia Seed Pudding with Fresh Fruit

Ingredients:

1/4 cup chia seeds

1 cup unsweetened almond milk

1 tablespoon honey or maple syrup

1/2 teaspoon vanilla extract

1/2 cup fresh fruit (mango, berries, kiwi)

Instructions:

1. In a bowl, mix chia seeds, almond milk, honey, and vanilla extract.

2. Stir well and let it sit for 5 minutes. Stir again to prevent clumping.

3. Cover and refrigerate for at least 2 hours or overnight.

4. Serve topped with fresh fruit for a refreshing and nutritious breakfast that supports healthy blood sugar levels.

10. Smoothie Bowl with Greens and Berries

Ingredients:

1 cup spinach or kale

1 frozen banana

1/2 cup mixed berries

1/2 cup unsweetened almond milk

1 tablespoon chia seeds

1 tablespoon almond butter

Toppings: granola, sliced almonds, fresh berries, coconut flakes

Instructions:

1. Blend spinach or kale, frozen banana, mixed berries, almond milk, chia seeds, and almond butter until smooth.

2. Pour into a bowl.

3. Top with granola, sliced almonds, fresh berries, and coconut flakes.

4. Enjoy a delicious, nutrient-dense bowl that helps maintain balanced blood sugar levels.

• **Healthy Takes on Traditional Breakfasts**

11. Almond Flour Pancakes

Ingredients:

1 cup almond flour

2 large eggs

1/4 cup unsweetened almond milk

1 teaspoon baking powder

1 teaspoon vanilla extract

1 tablespoon coconut oil (for cooking)

Fresh berries and a drizzle of honey for topping

Instructions:

1. In a bowl, whisk together almond flour, eggs, almond milk, baking powder, and vanilla extract until smooth.

2. Heat coconut oil in a non-stick skillet over medium heat.

3. Pour batter into the skillet to form small pancakes.

4. Cook for 2-3 minutes on each side until golden brown.

5. Serve with fresh berries and a drizzle of honey for a healthy, blood sugar-friendly breakfast.

12. Veggie-Packed Omelet

Ingredients:

3 large eggs

1/4 cup bell peppers, chopped

1/4 cup spinach, chopped

1/4 cup mushrooms, sliced

1/4 cup onion, chopped

1 tablespoon olive oil

Salt and pepper to taste

Instructions:

1. In a bowl, whisk the eggs with salt and pepper.

2. Heat olive oil in a skillet over medium heat.

3. Sauté bell peppers, spinach, mushrooms, and onion until tender.

4. Pour the eggs over the vegetables in the skillet.

5. Cook until the eggs are set, folding the omelet in half.

6. Serve hot for a filling, blood sugar-friendly start to your day.

13. Whole Grain Avocado Toast

Ingredients:

2 slices whole grain bread

1 ripe avocado

1/2 lemon, juiced

Salt and pepper to taste

Red pepper flakes (optional)

1 tablespoon chia seeds

Instructions:

1. Toast the whole grain bread slices to your preference.

2. In a bowl, mash the avocado with lemon juice, salt, and pepper.

3. Spread the avocado mixture evenly over the toast.

4. Sprinkle with red pepper flakes and chia seeds.

5. Enjoy a delicious and simple breakfast that supports healthy blood sugar levels.

13. Cottage Cheese and Fruit Bowl

Ingredients:

1 cup low-fat cottage cheese

1/2 cup fresh pineapple chunks

1/2 cup fresh berries

1 tablespoon chia seeds

1 tablespoon honey (optional)

Instructions:

1. Place the cottage cheese in a bowl.

2. Top with fresh pineapple chunks and berries.

3. Sprinkle chia seeds over the top.

4. Drizzle with honey if desired.

5. Enjoy this high-protein, blood sugar-friendly breakfast.

14. Sweet Potato and Egg Breakfast Hash

Ingredients:

1 large sweet potato, diced

1/2 onion, chopped

1/2 bell pepper, chopped

1 tablespoon olive oil

2 large eggs

Salt and pepper to taste

Fresh parsley, chopped (optional)

Instructions:

1. Heat olive oil in a skillet over medium heat.

2. Add diced sweet potato, onion, and bell pepper. Cook until tender, about 10 minutes.

3. Push the vegetables to the side of the skillet and crack the eggs into the empty space.

4. Cook until the eggs are done to your liking.

5. Season with salt and pepper, and garnish with fresh parsley if desired.

6. Serve hot for a nutritious and satisfying breakfast that keeps blood sugar stable.

Chapter 2

Lunch Recipes

• Satisfying Salads

15. Grilled Chicken and Avocado Salad

Ingredients:

2 grilled chicken breasts, sliced

1 ripe avocado, sliced

4 cups mixed greens (spinach, kale, arugula)

1 cup cherry tomatoes, halved

1/4 cup red onion, thinly sliced

1/4 cup feta cheese, crumbled

1/4 cup olive oil

2 tablespoons balsamic vinegar

Salt and pepper to taste

Instructions:

1. Place mixed greens in a large salad bowl.

2. Add the grilled chicken slices, avocado, cherry tomatoes, red onion, and feta cheese.

3. In a small bowl, whisk together the olive oil, balsamic vinegar, salt, and pepper.

4. Drizzle the dressing over the salad and toss gently to combine.

5. Serve immediately.

16. Spinach and Quinoa Salad with Citrus Dressing

Ingredients:

2 cups cooked quinoa

4 cups fresh spinach leaves

1/2 cup sliced almonds

1/2 cup dried cranberries

1/4 cup goat cheese, crumbled

1 orange, peeled and segmented

1/4 cup orange juice

2 tablespoons lemon juice

1/4 cup olive oil

Salt and pepper to taste

Instructions:

1. In a large bowl, combine the cooked quinoa and fresh spinach.

2. Add the sliced almonds, dried cranberries, goat cheese, and orange segments.

3. In a small bowl, whisk together the orange juice, lemon juice, olive oil, salt, and pepper.

4. Pour the dressing over the salad and toss well to coat.

5. Serve chilled.

• Hearty Soups and Stews

17. Lentil and Vegetable Soup

Ingredients:

1 cup lentils, rinsed

1 large onion, chopped

2 carrots, diced

2 celery stalks, chopped

3 garlic cloves, minced

1 can diced tomatoes (14.5 oz)

6 cups vegetable broth

2 teaspoons ground cumin

1 teaspoon smoked paprika

Salt and pepper to taste

2 tablespoons olive oil

Instructions:

1. In a large pot, heat olive oil over medium heat.

2. Add the onion, carrots, celery, and garlic. Sauté until vegetables are tender.

3. Stir in the lentils, diced tomatoes, vegetable broth, cumin, smoked paprika, salt, and pepper.

4. Bring to a boil, then reduce heat and simmer for 30-35 minutes, or until lentils are cooked.

5. Serve hot.

18. Chicken and Bean Stew

Ingredients:

2 chicken breasts, cubed

1 can white beans (15 oz), drained and rinsed

1 can diced tomatoes (14.5 oz)

1 large onion, chopped

2 cloves garlic, minced

1 red bell pepper, chopped

1 teaspoon dried oregano

1 teaspoon ground cumin

4 cups chicken broth

2 tablespoons olive oil

Salt and pepper to taste

Instructions:

1. Heat olive oil in a large pot over medium heat.

2. Add chicken and cook until browned. Remove and set aside.

3. In the same pot, sauté onion, garlic, and red bell pepper until softened.

4. Stir in diced tomatoes, white beans, chicken broth, oregano, cumin, salt, and pepper.

5. Return chicken to the pot and bring to a boil. Reduce heat and simmer for 25-30 minutes.

6. Serve warm.

● Balanced Sandwiches and Wraps

19. Turkey and Veggie Wrap

Ingredients:

1 whole wheat wrap

4 slices turkey breast

1/4 cup hummus

1/2 avocado, sliced

1/4 cup shredded carrots

1/4 cup baby spinach

Salt and pepper to taste

Instructions:

1. Spread hummus evenly over the whole wheat wrap.

2. Layer turkey slices, avocado, shredded carrots, and baby spinach on top.

3. Season with salt and pepper.

4. Roll up tightly and slice in half.

5. Serve immediately.

20. Tuna Salad on Whole Grain Bread

Ingredients:

2 slices whole grain bread

1 can tuna in water, drained

2 tablespoons Greek yogurt

1 tablespoon Dijon mustard

1 celery stalk, chopped

1 green onion, chopped

1/4 teaspoon black pepper

1/2 teaspoon lemon juice

Instructions:

1. In a bowl, mix tuna, Greek yogurt, Dijon mustard, celery, green onion, black pepper, and lemon juice.

2. Spread the tuna mixture evenly on one slice of whole grain bread.

3. Top with the second slice of bread.

4. Slice in half and serve.

21. Avocado and Chickpea Salad Sandwich

Ingredients:

2 slices whole grain bread

1 ripe avocado

1 cup canned chickpeas, drained and rinsed

1 tablespoon lemon juice

1 tablespoon tahini

1/2 teaspoon ground cumin

1/4 teaspoon salt

1/4 teaspoon black pepper

1/4 cup shredded lettuce

1/4 cup grated carrots

Instructions:

1. In a bowl, mash the avocado and chickpeas together until well combined.

2. Stir in lemon juice, tahini, ground cumin, salt, and black pepper.

3. Spread the avocado and chickpea mixture onto one slice of whole grain bread.

4. Top with shredded lettuce and grated carrots.

5. Place the second slice of bread on top, slice in half, and serve.

22. Grilled Veggie and Hummus Wrap

Ingredients:

1 whole wheat wrap

1/4 cup hummus

1/2 red bell pepper, sliced

1/2 zucchini, sliced

1/2 eggplant, sliced

1/4 cup crumbled feta cheese

1 tablespoon olive oil

1/4 teaspoon dried oregano

Salt and pepper to taste

Instructions:

1. Heat olive oil in a grill pan over medium heat.

2. Grill the red bell pepper, zucchini, and eggplant slices until tender and slightly charred.

3. Season with dried oregano, salt, and pepper.

4. Spread hummus evenly over the whole wheat wrap.

5. Layer the grilled veggies and sprinkle with crumbled feta cheese.

6. Roll up tightly and slice in half.

7. Serve warm or at room temperature.

23. Chicken Caesar Wrap

Ingredients:

1 whole wheat wrap

1 grilled chicken breast, sliced

1 cup romaine lettuce, chopped

1/4 cup Caesar dressing (preferably low-fat)

2 tablespoons grated Parmesan cheese

1/4 cup cherry tomatoes, halved

Instructions:

1. In a bowl, toss the chopped romaine lettuce with Caesar dressing until well coated.

2. Lay the whole wheat wrap flat and place the sliced grilled chicken in the center.

3. Add the dressed romaine lettuce, grated Parmesan cheese, and cherry tomatoes on top of the chicken.

4. Roll up tightly and slice in half.

5. Serve immediately.

These recipes are designed to keep your blood sugar levels stable while providing delicious, balanced meals. They are easy to prepare, packed with nutrients, and perfect for anyone looking to maintain a healthy diet.

Chapter 3

Dinner Recipes

● Protein-Rich Main Dishes

24. Baked Salmon with Asparagus

Ingredients:

4 salmon fillets

1 bunch asparagus, trimmed

2 tablespoons olive oil

Salt and pepper to taste

Lemon slices for garnish

Instructions:

1. Preheat the oven to 375°F (190°C).

2. Place the salmon fillets on a baking sheet lined with parchment paper.

3. Arrange the asparagus around the salmon.

4. Drizzle olive oil over the salmon and asparagus, then season with salt and pepper.

5. Bake for 12-15 minutes, or until the salmon is cooked through and flakes easily with a fork.

6. Serve hot, garnished with lemon slices.

25. Garlic Herb Chicken Breasts

Ingredients:

4 boneless, skinless chicken breasts

4 cloves garlic, minced

2 tablespoons olive oil

1 teaspoon dried thyme

1 teaspoon dried rosemary

Salt and pepper to taste

Instructions:

1. Preheat the oven to 400°F (200°C).

2. In a small bowl, mix together the minced garlic, olive oil, thyme, rosemary, salt, and pepper.

3. Place the chicken breasts in a baking dish and coat them with the garlic herb mixture.

4. Bake for 20-25 minutes, or until the chicken is cooked through and juices run clear.

5. Serve hot with your favorite side dishes.

26. Grilled Steak with Roasted Vegetables

Ingredients:

4 beef steak cuts (such as sirloin or ribeye)

2 bell peppers, sliced

1 red onion, sliced

2 tablespoons olive oil

Salt and pepper to taste

Instructions:

1. Preheat the grill to medium-high heat.

2. Season the steak cuts with salt and pepper on both sides.

3. In a bowl, toss the sliced peppers and onion with olive oil, salt, and pepper.

4. Grill the steak for 4-6 minutes per side, depending on desired doneness.

5. Meanwhile, spread the seasoned vegetables on a baking sheet and roast in the oven at 400°F (200°C) for 15-20 minutes, or until tender.

6. Serve the grilled steak with roasted vegetables on the side.

27. Turkey Meatballs in Marinara Sauce

Ingredients:

1 lb ground turkey

1/4 cup breadcrumbs

1/4 cup grated Parmesan cheese

1 egg

1 teaspoon dried oregano

1 teaspoon dried basil

Salt and pepper to taste

2 cups marinara sauce

Instructions:

1. Preheat the oven to 375°F (190°C).

2. In a large bowl, combine the ground turkey, breadcrumbs, Parmesan cheese, egg, oregano, basil, salt, and pepper. Mix until well combined.

3. Shape the mixture into meatballs and place them on a baking sheet lined with parchment paper.

4. Bake for 20-25 minutes, or until the meatballs are cooked through.

5. Heat the marinara sauce in a saucepan over medium heat. Add the cooked meatballs to the sauce and simmer for 5-10 minutes.

6. Serve hot over cooked pasta or with crusty bread.

28. Tofu Stir-Fry with Vegetables

Ingredients:

1 block extra-firm tofu, pressed and cubed

2 cups mixed vegetables (such as bell peppers, broccoli, carrots)

2 tablespoons soy sauce

1 tablespoon sesame oil

2 cloves garlic, minced

1 teaspoon ginger, grated

Cooked brown rice for serving

Instructions:

1. Heat sesame oil in a large skillet over medium heat. Add garlic and ginger, sauté for 1 minute.

2. Add tofu cubes to the skillet and cook until golden brown on all sides.

3. Add mixed vegetables and soy sauce to the skillet. Stir-fry for 5-7 minutes, or until vegetables are tender-crisp.

4. Serve hot over cooked brown rice.

• Flavorful Veggie Sides

29. Roasted Brussels Sprouts

Ingredients:

1 lb Brussels sprouts, trimmed and halved

2 tablespoons olive oil

Salt and pepper to taste

Instructions:

1. Preheat the oven to 400°F (200°C).

2. Toss Brussels sprouts with olive oil, salt, and pepper in a bowl until evenly coated.

3. Spread the Brussels sprouts in a single layer on a baking sheet.

4. Roast for 20-25 minutes, or until tender and caramelized, stirring halfway through cooking.

5. Serve hot as a side dish.

30. Cauliflower Mash

Ingredients:

1 head cauliflower, chopped into florets

2 cloves garlic, minced

2 tablespoons butter

Salt and pepper to taste

Chopped chives for garnish (optional)

Instructions:

1. Steam or boil cauliflower florets until tender, about 10-12 minutes.

2. Drain the cauliflower and transfer it to a food processor.

3. Add minced garlic, butter, salt, and pepper to the food processor.

4. Blend until smooth and creamy, scraping down the sides as needed.

5. Transfer the cauliflower mash to a serving bowl, garnish with chopped chives if desired, and serve hot.

31. Sautéed Garlic Spinach

Ingredients:

1 lb fresh spinach leaves

2 cloves garlic, minced

1 tablespoon olive oil

Salt and pepper to taste

Lemon wedges for serving (optional)

Instructions:

1. Heat olive oil in a large skillet over medium heat.

2. Add minced garlic to the skillet and sauté for 1 minute until fragrant.

3. Add fresh spinach leaves to the skillet and toss to coat with garlic oil.

4. Cook spinach for 2-3 minutes, stirring occasionally, until wilted.

5. Season with salt and pepper to taste.

6. Serve hot with a squeeze of lemon juice if desired.

32. Grilled Vegetables

Ingredients:

Assorted vegetables (such as zucchini, bell peppers, eggplant, mushrooms)

2 tablespoons olive oil

Salt and pepper to taste

Fresh herbs for garnish (optional)

Instructions:

1. Preheat the grill to medium-high heat.

2. Slice the vegetables into even-sized pieces.

3. Toss the vegetables with olive oil, salt, and pepper in a bowl until evenly coated.

4. Grill the vegetables for 5-7 minutes per side, or until tender and grill marks appear.

5. Remove from the grill and garnish with fresh herbs if desired.

6. Serve hot as a side dish or as part of a grilled vegetable platter.

33. Steamed Broccoli with Garlic Butter

Ingredients:

1 lb broccoli florets

2 tablespoons butter

2 cloves garlic, minced

Salt and pepper to taste

Lemon wedges for serving (optional)

Instructions:

1. Steam broccoli florets until tender, about 5-7 minutes.

2. In a small saucepan, melt butter over medium heat.

3. Add minced garlic to the melted butter and sauté for 1 minute until fragrant.

4. Drizzle the garlic butter over the steamed broccoli.

5. Season with salt and pepper to taste.

6. Serve hot with lemon wedges on the side if desired.

• **Whole-Grain Comfort Foods**

34. Brown Rice Stir-Fry

Ingredients:

2 cups cooked brown rice

1 cup mixed vegetables (such as bell peppers, carrots, broccoli)

1 tablespoon sesame oil

2 cloves garlic, minced

2 tablespoons soy sauce

1 tablespoon rice vinegar

1 teaspoon grated ginger

Sesame seeds for garnish (optional)

Instructions:

1. Heat sesame oil in a large skillet or wok over medium-high heat.

2. Add minced garlic and grated ginger to the skillet and sauté for 1 minute.

3. Add mixed vegetables to the skillet and stir-fry for 3-4 minutes, until crisp-tender.

4. Stir in cooked brown rice, soy sauce, and rice vinegar, and cook for an additional 2-3 minutes, until heated through.

5. Garnish with sesame seeds if desired and serve hot.

35. Quinoa Stuffed Peppers

Ingredients:

4 large bell peppers, halved and seeds removed

1 cup quinoa, cooked

1 can (15 oz) black beans, drained and rinsed

1 cup corn kernels

1 cup diced tomatoes

1 teaspoon chili powder

1/2 teaspoon cumin

Salt and pepper to taste

Shredded cheese for topping (optional)

Instructions:

1. Preheat the oven to 375°F (190°C).

2. In a large bowl, mix together cooked quinoa, black beans, corn kernels, diced tomatoes, chili powder, cumin, salt, and pepper.

3. Stuff each bell pepper half with the quinoa mixture.

4. Place the stuffed peppers in a baking dish and cover with foil.

5. Bake for 25-30 minutes, or until the peppers are tender.

6. If desired, sprinkle shredded cheese on top of the peppers during the last 5 minutes of baking.

7. Serve hot as a comforting and nutritious meal.

36. Whole Wheat Pasta Primavera

Ingredients:

8 oz whole wheat pasta

2 tablespoons olive oil

2 cloves garlic, minced

1 cup mixed vegetables (such as bell peppers, zucchini, cherry tomatoes)

1/2 cup grated Parmesan cheese

Salt and pepper to taste

Fresh basil leaves for garnish (optional)

Instructions:

1. Cook whole wheat pasta according to package instructions until al dente. Drain and set aside.

2. Heat olive oil in a large skillet over medium heat. Add minced garlic and sauté for 1 minute.

3. Add mixed vegetables to the skillet and cook for 5-7 minutes, until tender.

4. Toss cooked pasta with the vegetable mixture in the skillet.

5. Stir in grated Parmesan cheese and season with salt and pepper to taste.

6. Garnish with fresh basil leaves if desired and serve hot.

36. Quinoa and Black Bean Chili

Ingredients:

1 cup quinoa, rinsed

1 can (15 oz) black beans, drained and rinsed

1 can (15 oz) diced tomatoes

1 bell pepper, diced

1 onion, diced

2 cloves garlic, minced

2 tablespoons chili powder

1 teaspoon cumin

Salt and pepper to taste

Chopped cilantro for garnish (optional)

Instructions:

1. In a large pot, heat olive oil over medium heat. Add diced onion and bell pepper, and sauté until softened.

2. Add minced garlic, chili powder, and cumin to the pot, and cook for 1 minute until fragrant.

3. Stir in quinoa, black beans, diced tomatoes, and 3 cups of water. Bring to a boil.

4. Reduce heat to low, cover, and simmer for 20-25 minutes, or until quinoa is cooked and chili has thickened.

5. Season with salt and pepper to taste.

6. Serve hot, garnished with chopped cilantro if desired.

37. Sweet Potato and Black Bean Enchiladas

Ingredients:

1 large sweet potato, peeled and diced

1 can (15 oz) black beans, drained and rinsed

1 bell pepper, diced

1 onion, diced

2 cloves garlic, minced

1 teaspoon chili powder

1/2 teaspoon cumin

8 whole wheat tortillas

1 cup enchilada sauce

1/2 cup shredded cheese (such as cheddar or Monterey Jack)

Chopped cilantro for garnish (optional)

Instructions:

1. Preheat the oven to 375°F (190°C).

2. In a large skillet, heat olive oil over medium heat. Add diced sweet potato, bell pepper, onion, and minced garlic, and sauté until vegetables are tender.

3. Stir in black beans, chili powder, and cumin, and cook for an additional 2-3 minutes.

4. Spoon the sweet potato and black bean mixture onto each whole wheat tortilla, roll up, and place seam-side down in a baking dish.

5. Pour enchilada sauce over the rolled tortillas and sprinkle with shredded cheese.

6. Cover the baking dish with foil and bake for 20-25 minutes, or until heated through and cheese is melted.

7. Garnish with chopped cilantro if desired and serve hot.

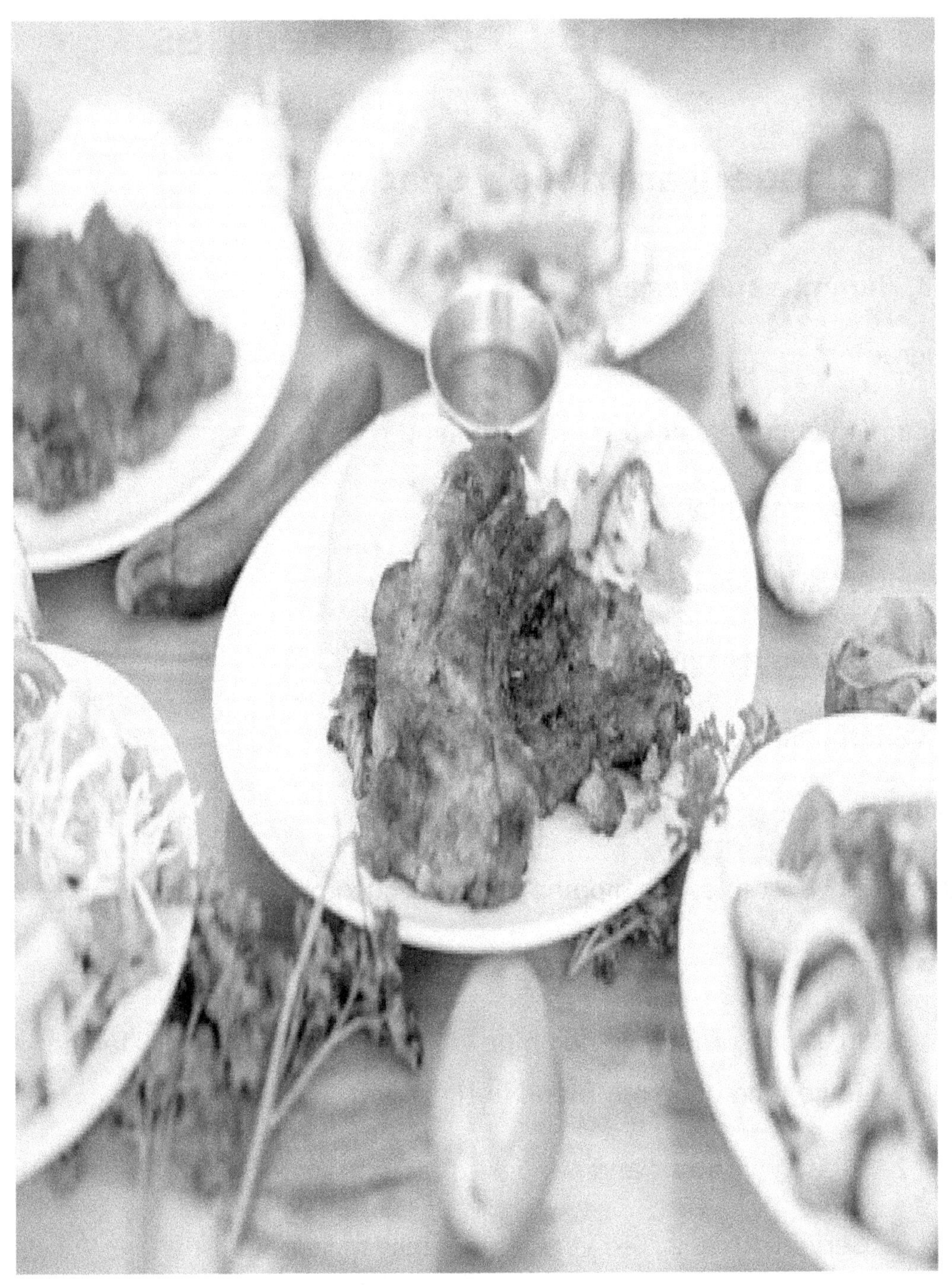

Chapter 4

Snack and Dessert Recipes

● Blood Sugar-Friendly Snacks

38. Hummus and Veggie Sticks

Ingredients:

1 can (15 ounces) chickpeas, drained and rinsed

2 tablespoons tahini

2 cloves garlic, minced

2 tablespoons lemon juice

2 tablespoons olive oil

Salt and pepper to taste

Assorted vegetables for dipping (carrots, cucumbers, bell peppers)

Instructions:

1. In a food processor, combine chickpeas, tahini, garlic, lemon juice, and olive oil. Blend until smooth.

2. Season with salt and pepper to taste.

3. Serve with assorted vegetable sticks for dipping.

39. Nut Mix with Dark Chocolate Chips

Ingredients:

1 cup mixed nuts (almonds, walnuts, cashews)

¼ cup dark chocolate chips

Instructions:

1. In a bowl, mix together mixed nuts and dark chocolate chips.

2. Portion into small snack bags for easy grab-and-go access.

40. Greek Yogurt with Berries

Ingredients:

1 cup Greek yogurt

½ cup mixed berries (strawberries, blueberries, raspberries)

1 tablespoon honey (optional)

Instructions:

1. Spoon Greek yogurt into a bowl.

2. Top with mixed berries and drizzle with honey if desired.

41. Avocado Toast with Tomato

Ingredients:

2 slices whole grain bread

1 ripe avocado

1 small tomato, sliced

Salt and pepper to taste

Instructions:

1. Toast the whole grain bread slices until golden brown.

2. Mash the ripe avocado and spread it evenly on the toasted bread.

3. Top with sliced tomato and season with salt and pepper.

42. Apple Slices with Almond Butter

Ingredients:

1 apple, cored and sliced

2 tablespoons almond butter

Instructions:

1. Spread almond butter on apple slices.

2. Enjoy as a satisfying and crunchy snack.

● Guilt-Free Desserts

43. Chia Seed Pudding

Ingredients:

¼ cup chia seeds

1 cup almond milk

1 tablespoon maple syrup

½ teaspoon vanilla extract

Instructions:

1. In a bowl, mix together chia seeds, almond milk, maple syrup, and vanilla extract.

2. Refrigerate for at least 2 hours or overnight until the pudding thickens.

3. Serve with fresh fruit toppings if desired.

44. Berry and Greek Yogurt Parfait

Ingredients:

1 cup Greek yogurt

½ cup mixed berries (strawberries, blueberries, raspberries)

2 tablespoons granola

Instructions:

1. Layer Greek yogurt, mixed berries, and granola in a glass.

2. Repeat layers until the glass is filled.

3. Serve immediately as a refreshing dessert or snack.

45. Banana Nice Cream

Ingredients:

2 ripe bananas, sliced and frozen

2 tablespoons cocoa powder

1 tablespoon honey (optional)

Instructions:

1. In a blender, combine frozen banana slices, cocoa powder, and honey (if using).

2. Blend until smooth and creamy.

3. Serve immediately as a healthy alternative to ice cream.

46. Coconut Date Energy Balls

Ingredients:

1 cup Medjool dates, pitted

1 cup unsweetened shredded coconut

¼ cup almonds

1 tablespoon coconut oil

Instructions:

1. In a food processor, combine dates, shredded coconut, almonds, and coconut oil.

2. Pulse until mixture forms a sticky dough.

3. Roll into small balls and refrigerate until firm.

47. Frozen Yogurt Bark

Ingredients:

2 cups Greek yogurt

½ cup mixed berries (strawberries, blueberries, raspberries)

2 tablespoons honey

Instructions:

1. Line a baking sheet with parchment paper.

2. Spread Greek yogurt evenly onto the parchment paper.

3. Sprinkle mixed berries and drizzle honey over the yogurt.

4. Freeze for 2-3 hours until firm.

5. Break into pieces and enjoy as a refreshing dessert.

• Healthy Baking

48. Almond Flour Cookies

Ingredients:

2 cups almond flour

1 egg

¼ cup honey

1 teaspoon vanilla extract

¼ teaspoon baking soda

Pinch of salt

Instructions:

1. Preheat the oven to 350°F (175°C) and line a baking sheet with parchment paper.

2. In a bowl, mix together almond flour, egg, honey, vanilla extract, baking soda, and salt until a dough forms.

3. Roll the dough into balls and place them on the prepared baking sheet.

4. Flatten the balls with a fork and bake for 10-12 minutes until golden brown.

5. Allow to cool before serving.

49. Zucchini Bread

Ingredients:

2 cups grated zucchini

2 cups whole wheat flour

½ cup honey

½ cup unsweetened applesauce

2 eggs

1 teaspoon vanilla extract

1 teaspoon cinnamon

½ teaspoon baking powder

½ teaspoon baking soda

Pinch of salt

Instructions:

1. Preheat the oven to 350°F (175°C) and grease a loaf pan.

2. In a large bowl, mix together grated zucchini, whole wheat flour, honey, applesauce, eggs, vanilla extract, cinnamon, baking powder, baking soda, and salt until well combined.

3. Pour the batter into the prepared loaf pan and bake for 50-60 minutes until a toothpick inserted into the center comes out clean.

4. Allow the zucchini bread to cool before slicing and serving.

50. Oatmeal Raisin Cookies

Ingredients:

1 cup rolled oats

½ cup almond flour

½ cup raisins

¼ cup coconut oil, melted

¼ cup maple syrup

1 egg

1 teaspoon vanilla extract

½ teaspoon cinnamon

Pinch of salt

Instructions:

1. Preheat the oven to 350°F (175°C) and line a baking sheet with parchment paper.

2. In a bowl, mix together rolled oats, almond flour, raisins, melted coconut oil, maple syrup, egg, vanilla extract, cinnamon, and salt until well combined.

3. Drop spoonfuls of the cookie dough onto the prepared baking sheet.

4. Bake for 12-15 minutes until the edges are golden brown.

5. Allow the cookies to cool on the baking sheet before transferring to a wire rack.

51. Peanut Butter Banana Bites

Ingredients:

2 ripe bananas, sliced

¼ cup natural peanut butter

¼ cup granola

Instructions:

1. Spread peanut butter on one side of each banana slice.

2. Sprinkle granola over half of the banana slices.

3. Top with the remaining banana slices to make sandwiches.

4. Serve immediately or freeze for a refreshing treat.

52. Carrot Cake Muffins

Ingredients:

1 ½ cups whole wheat flour

1 cup grated carrots

½ cup chopped walnuts

½ cup raisins

⅓ cup honey

⅓ cup unsweetened applesauce

2 eggs

¼ cup coconut oil, melted

1 teaspoon vanilla extract

1 teaspoon cinnamon

½ teaspoon baking powder

½ teaspoon baking soda

Pinch of salt

Instructions:

1. Preheat the oven to 350°F (175°C) and line a muffin tin with paper liners.

2. In a large bowl, mix together whole wheat flour, grated carrots, chopped walnuts, raisins, honey, applesauce, eggs, melted coconut oil, vanilla extract, cinnamon, baking powder, baking soda, and salt until well combined.

3. Spoon the batter into the prepared muffin tin, filling each cup about ¾ full.

4. Bake for 20-25 minutes until a toothpick inserted into the center comes out clean.

5. Allow the muffins to cool in the tin for 5 minutes before transferring to a wire rack to cool completely.

Chapter 5

Drinks and Smoothies

- **Refreshing Beverages**

53. Lemon and Mint Water

Ingredients:

1 lemon, sliced

Handful of fresh mint leaves

Ice cubes

Water

Instructions:

1. Fill a pitcher with water.

2. Add lemon slices and mint leaves.

3. Stir well and let it sit in the refrigerator for at least 30 minutes to allow flavors to infuse.

4. Serve over ice and garnish with additional mint leaves if desired.

54. Herbal Teas

Ingredients:

- Herbal tea bags (such as chamomile, peppermint, or cinnamon)

- Water

- **Optional:** honey or stevia for sweetness

Instructions:

1. Boil water in a kettle or pot.

2. Place herbal tea bag in a mug.

3. Pour hot water over the tea bag and let it steep for 5-7 minutes.

4. Remove the tea bag and add sweetener if desired.

5. Stir well and enjoy your soothing herbal tea.

• Blood Sugar-Balancing Smoothies

55. Green Detox Smoothie

Ingredients:

1 cup spinach

1/2 cucumber, peeled and chopped

1/2 green apple, cored and chopped

1/2 lemon, juiced

1/2 inch piece of ginger, peeled

1/2 cup coconut water

Ice cubes

Instructions:

1. Place all ingredients in a blender.

2. Blend until smooth and creamy.

3. Add more coconut water if needed for desired consistency.

4. Pour into glasses and serve immediately.

56. Berry Protein Smoothie

Ingredients:

1/2 cup mixed berries (such as strawberries, blueberries, and raspberries)

1/2 banana, frozen

1/2 cup plain Greek yogurt

1 scoop vanilla protein powder

1 tablespoon chia seeds

1 cup almond milk

Ice cubes

Instructions:

1. Combine all ingredients in a blender.

2. Blend until smooth and creamy.

3. Add more almond milk if needed for desired consistency.

4. Pour into glasses and enjoy your protein-packed berry smoothie.

57. Avocado and Kale Smoothie

Ingredients:

1/2 ripe avocado

1 cup kale leaves, stems removed

1/2 green apple, cored and chopped

1 tablespoon chia seeds

1 cup unsweetened almond milk

1/2 cup water

Ice cubes (optional)

Instructions:

1. Place avocado, kale, green apple, chia seeds, almond milk, and water in a blender.

2. Blend until smooth and creamy.

3. Add ice cubes if desired and blend again until well combined.

4. Pour into glasses and serve immediately.

58. Tropical Turmeric Smoothie

Ingredients:

1/2 cup pineapple chunks

1/2 cup mango chunks

1 small carrot, peeled and chopped

1/2 teaspoon ground turmeric

1 tablespoon flaxseed oil

1 cup coconut water

Ice cubes (optional)

Instructions:

1. Combine pineapple, mango, carrot, turmeric, flaxseed oil, and coconut water in a blender.

2. Blend until smooth and creamy.

3. Add ice cubes if desired and blend again until well combined.

4. Pour into glasses and enjoy this anti-inflammatory, blood sugar-friendly smoothie.

59. Cinnamon Almond Smoothie

Ingredients:

1/2 cup unsweetened almond milk

1/2 banana

1 tablespoon almond butter

1/2 teaspoon ground cinnamon

1 tablespoon chia seeds

1/2 teaspoon vanilla extract

Ice cubes (optional)

Instructions:

1. In a blender, combine almond milk, banana, almond butter, cinnamon, chia seeds, and vanilla extract.

2. Blend until smooth and creamy.

3. Add ice cubes if desired and blend again until well combined.

4. Pour into glasses and serve immediately.

60. Blueberry Spinach Smoothie

Ingredients:

1/2 cup fresh or frozen blueberries

1 cup spinach leaves

1/2 banana

1/2 cup Greek yogurt

1 tablespoon hemp seeds

1 cup unsweetened almond milk

Ice cubes (optional)

Instructions:

1. Place blueberries, spinach, banana, Greek yogurt, hemp seeds, and almond milk in a blender.

2. Blend until smooth and creamy.

3. Add ice cubes if desired and blend again until well combined.

4. Pour into glasses and enjoy this nutrient-packed, blood sugar-balancing smoothie.

Drinking these refreshing beverages and blood sugar-balancing smoothies daily will help you stay hydrated. It will also support your overall health while managing your blood sugar levels naturally.

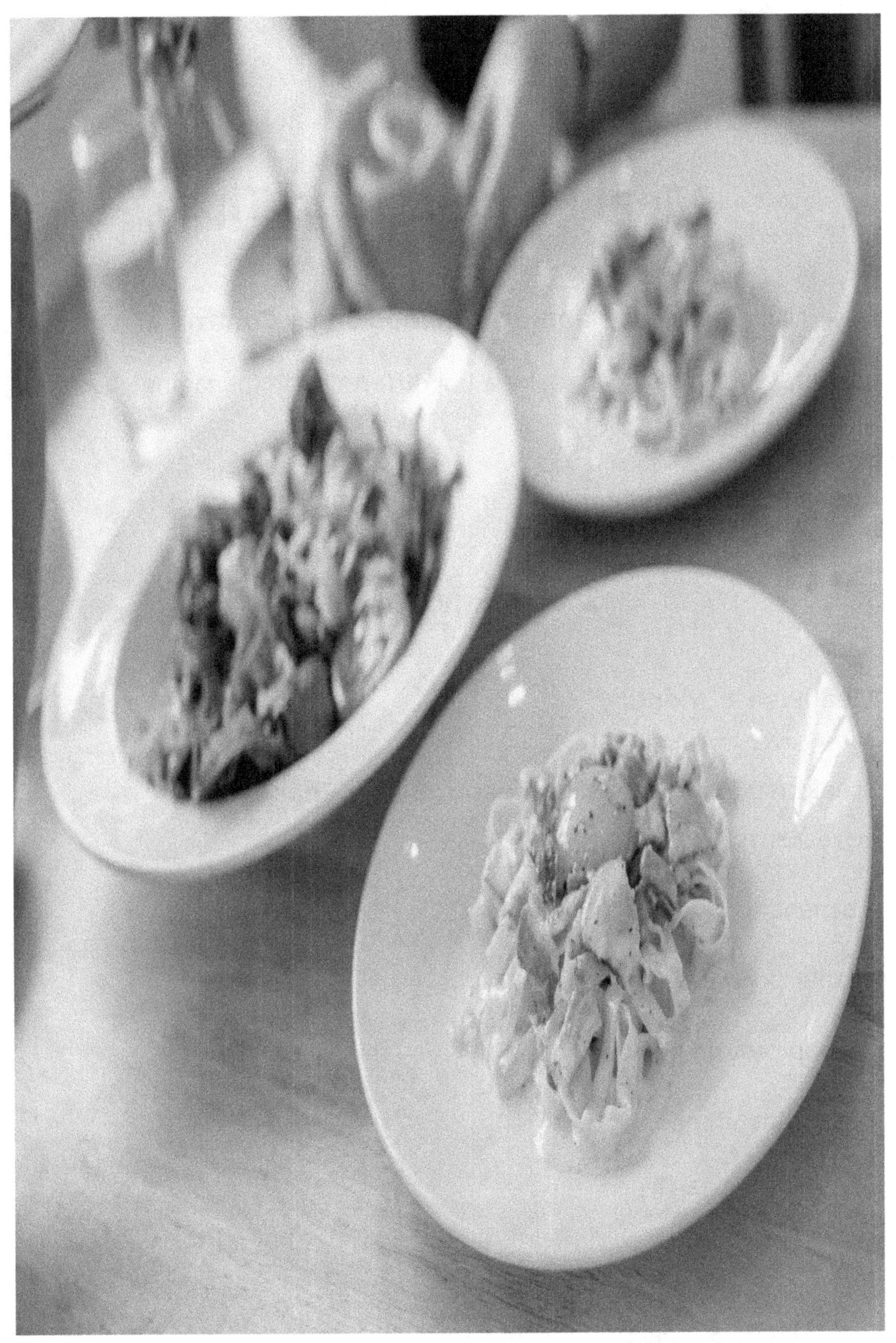

Chapter 6

Meal Planning and Tips

- **Weekly Meal Planning for Blood Sugar Control**

Planning your meals can make a big difference in managing your blood sugar levels.

Here are some sample meal plans to help you get started.

1 Week Meal Plan

Meal Plan 1: Monday

Breakfast: Protein-Packed Peanut Butter Shake
Ingredients:

1 banana

1 tablespoon peanut butter

1 scoop protein powder

1 cup almond milk

Ice cubes (optional)

Instructions:

1. Blend all ingredients until smooth.

2. Serve and enjoy!

Lunch: Grilled Chicken and Avocado Salad

Ingredients:

1 grilled chicken breast

Mixed greens

Cherry tomatoes

1/2 avocado

Balsamic vinaigrette dressing

Instructions:

1. Chop chicken and avocado.

2. Toss all ingredients together with dressing.

3. Serve chilled.

Dinner: Baked Salmon with Asparagus

Ingredients:

2 salmon fillets

1 bunch asparagus

Olive oil

Lemon slices

Salt and pepper to taste

Instructions:

1. Preheat oven to 400°F (200°C).

2. Place salmon and asparagus on a baking sheet.

3. Drizzle with olive oil and season with salt, pepper, and lemon slices.

4. Bake for 15-20 minutes or until salmon is cooked through.

5. Serve hot.

Meal Plan 2: Tuesday

Breakfast: Quinoa and Fruit Bowl

Ingredients:

1/2 cup cooked quinoa

Mixed berries

1 tablespoon honey

Almonds (optional)

Instructions:

1. Mix cooked quinoa with berries.

2. Drizzle with honey and sprinkle with almonds if desired.

3. Serve warm or chilled.

Lunch: Lentil and Vegetable Soup

Ingredients:

1 cup lentils

Mixed vegetables (carrots, celery, onion)

Vegetable broth

Salt and pepper to taste

Instructions:

1. In a pot, combine lentils, vegetables, and broth.

2. Season with salt and pepper.

3. Simmer for 20-25 minutes until lentils are tender.

4. Serve hot.

Dinner: Garlic Herb Chicken Breasts

Ingredients:

2 chicken breasts

Garlic cloves

Fresh herbs (rosemary, thyme)

Olive oil

Salt and pepper to taste

Instructions:

1. Preheat oven to 375°F (190°C).

2. Rub chicken with minced garlic, herbs, olive oil, salt, and pepper.

3. Bake for 25-30 minutes or until chicken is cooked through.

4. Serve with steamed vegetables.

Meal Plan 3: Wednesday

Breakfast: Almond Flour Pancakes

Ingredients:

1 cup almond flour

2 eggs

1/4 cup almond milk

1 tablespoon honey

1/2 teaspoon baking powder

1/2 teaspoon vanilla extract

Instructions:

1. In a bowl, whisk together almond flour, eggs, almond milk, honey, baking powder, and vanilla extract until smooth.

2. Heat a non-stick skillet over medium heat and lightly grease with oil.

3. Pour batter onto the skillet to form pancakes.

4. Cook until bubbles form on the surface, then flip and cook until golden brown.

5. Serve warm with your favorite toppings.

Lunch: Spinach and Quinoa Salad with Citrus Dressing

Ingredients:

1 cup cooked quinoa

Baby spinach

Orange segments

Toasted almonds

Citrus vinaigrette dressing

Instructions:

1. Toss cooked quinoa, spinach, orange segments, and toasted almonds together.

2. Drizzle with citrus vinaigrette dressing.

3. Serve chilled.

Dinner: Brown Rice Stir-Fry

Ingredients:

1 cup cooked brown rice

Mixed vegetables (bell peppers, broccoli, carrots)

Tofu or chicken

Soy sauce

Garlic powder

Sesame oil

Instructions:

1. In a pan, stir-fry tofu or chicken with mixed vegetables until cooked through.

2. Add cooked brown rice and season with soy sauce, garlic powder, and sesame oil.

3. Cook for another 2-3 minutes, stirring continuously.

4. Serve hot.

Meal Plan 4: Thursday

Breakfast: Veggie-Packed Omelet

Ingredients:

2 eggs

Mixed vegetables (bell peppers, onions, spinach)

Cheese (optional)

Salt and pepper to taste

Instructions:

1. In a bowl, beat eggs and season with salt and pepper.

2. Heat a non-stick skillet over medium heat and pour in beaten eggs.

3. Add mixed vegetables and cheese (if using) to one side of the omelet.

4. Fold the other side over the filling and cook until eggs are set.

5. Serve hot with a side of fresh fruit.

Lunch: Turkey and Veggie Wrap

Ingredients:

Whole grain tortilla

Sliced turkey breast

Hummus

Mixed greens

Sliced cucumber and tomato

Instructions:

1. Spread hummus on the tortilla.

2. Layer sliced turkey, mixed greens, cucumber, and tomato on top.

3. Roll up the tortilla tightly.

4. Slice in half and serve.

Dinner: Quinoa Stuffed Peppers

Ingredients:

Bell peppers

Cooked quinoa

Black beans

Corn kernels

Diced tomatoes

Taco seasoning

Shredded cheese (optional)

Instructions:

1. Preheat oven to 375°F (190°C).

2. Cut tops off bell peppers and remove seeds and membranes.

3. In a bowl, mix cooked quinoa, black beans, corn, diced tomatoes, and taco seasoning.

4. Stuff mixture into bell peppers and place in a baking dish.

5. Cover with foil and bake for 25-30 minutes.

6. Remove foil, sprinkle with cheese if desired, and bake for an additional 5 minutes until cheese is melted.

7. Serve hot.

Meal Plan 5: Friday

Breakfast: Greek Yogurt Parfait with Nuts

Ingredients:

Greek yogurt

Mixed berries

Granola

Chopped nuts (almonds, walnuts)

Honey (optional)

Instructions:

1. Layer Greek yogurt, mixed berries, granola, and chopped nuts in a glass or bowl.

2. Drizzle with honey if desired.

3. Serve chilled.

Lunch: Tuna Salad on Whole Grain Bread

Ingredients:

Canned tuna

Greek yogurt or mayo

Diced celery and onion

Dijon mustard

Whole grain bread

Lettuce and tomato slices

Instructions:

1. In a bowl, mix canned tuna, Greek yogurt or mayo, diced celery, onion, and Dijon mustard.

2. Spread tuna salad on whole grain bread slices.

3. Top with lettuce and tomato slices.

4. Serve as a sandwich.

Dinner: Zucchini Bread

Ingredients:

Grated zucchini

Whole wheat flour

Eggs

Greek yogurt

Honey

Cinnamon and nutmeg

Instructions:

1. Preheat oven to 350°F (175°C) and grease a loaf pan.

2. In a bowl, mix grated zucchini, whole wheat flour, eggs, Greek yogurt, honey, cinnamon, and nutmeg until well combined.

3. Pour batter into the loaf pan and smooth the top.

4. Bake for 50-60 minutes or until a toothpick inserted into the center comes out clean.

5. Let cool before slicing and serving.

Meal Plan 6: Saturday

Breakfast: Chia Seed Pudding

Ingredients:

Chia seeds

Almond milk

Vanilla extract

Honey or maple syrup

Fresh fruit for topping

Instructions:

1. In a jar or bowl, mix chia seeds, almond milk, vanilla extract, and sweetener.

2. Stir well and refrigerate overnight or for at least 4 hours until thickened.

3. Serve chilled with fresh fruit on top.

Lunch: Hummus and Veggie Sticks

Ingredients:

Hummus

Carrot, cucumber, and bell pepper sticks

Instructions:

1. Cut carrots, cucumber, and bell peppers into sticks.

2. Serve with hummus for dipping.

Dinner: Berry and Greek Yogurt Parfait

Ingredients:

Greek yogurt

Mixed berries

Granola

Honey (optional)

Instructions:

1. Layer Greek yogurt, mixed berries, and granola in a glass or bowl.

2. Drizzle with honey if desired.

3. Serve chilled.

Meal Plan 7: Sunday

Breakfast: Berry Protein Smoothie

Ingredients:

Mixed berries

Protein powder

Greek yogurt

Almond milk

Ice cubes

Instructions:

1. In a blender, combine mixed berries, protein powder, Greek yogurt, almond milk, and ice cubes.

2. Blend until smooth and creamy.

3. Pour into glasses and serve immediately.

Lunch: Grilled Chicken and Vegetable Skewers

Ingredients:

Chicken breast, cut into chunks

Bell peppers, onions, and zucchini, cut into chunks

Olive oil

Garlic powder

Salt and pepper to taste

Instructions:

1. Preheat grill to medium-high heat.

2. Thread chicken and vegetables onto skewers.

3. Drizzle with olive oil and season with garlic powder, salt, and pepper.

4. Grill skewers for 10-12 minutes, turning occasionally, until chicken is cooked through and vegetables are tender.

5. Serve hot with a side salad.

Dinner: Cauliflower Fried Rice

Ingredients:

Cauliflower rice

Mixed vegetables (peas, carrots, corn)

Eggs

Soy sauce

Sesame oil

Green onions for garnish

Instructions:

1. In a pan, stir-fry cauliflower rice and mixed vegetables until tender.

2. Push the rice mixture to one side of the pan and scramble eggs on the other side.

3. Once eggs are cooked, combine with the rice mixture.

4. Season with soy sauce and sesame oil to taste.

5. Garnish with chopped green onions before serving.

With these delicious and balanced meal plans, you can keep your blood sugar levels in check while enjoying a variety of flavorful dishes throughout the week.

Cooking Tips and Techniques

Cooking nutritious and delicious meals doesn't have to be complicated.

Below are some helpful tips and techniques to make your blood sugar-friendly cooking experience enjoyable and successful.

- **Healthier Cooking Methods**

i. **Grilling:** Grilling is a fantastic way to cook lean proteins like chicken, fish, and vegetables without adding extra fats or oils. The high heat seals in flavor and creates delicious char marks, enhancing the taste of your dishes.

ii. **Steaming:** Steaming vegetables preserves their natural nutrients and vibrant colors. It's a quick and easy method that retains moisture and results in tender, crisp veggies perfect for salads, stir-fries, or side dishes.

iii. **Baking:** Baking is a versatile cooking method that allows you to create a wide range of blood sugar-friendly dishes. From baked chicken breasts and fish fillets to roasted vegetables and homemade granola, the oven can do it all with minimal added fats.

iv. **Stir-Frying:** Stir-frying involves cooking ingredients quickly over high heat in a small amount of oil. It's a popular method in Asian cuisine and works well for combining lean proteins, colorful vegetables, and flavorful sauces in one pan for a balanced meal.

v. **Sauteing**: Sauteing is similar to stir-frying but typically involves cooking ingredients in a skillet over medium heat with a bit more oil. It's great for cooking delicate proteins like shrimp or tofu and quickly softening vegetables for pasta dishes or grain bowls.

- **Flavor-Boosting Tips**

i. **Herbs and Spices**: Experiment with a variety of herbs and spices to add flavor to your dishes without relying on salt or sugar. From aromatic garlic and ginger to bold cumin and paprika, there are endless combinations to enhance your meals.

ii. **Citrus Zest**: Don't toss those citrus peels! Grate or zest lemon, lime, or orange peels to infuse your recipes with bright, tangy flavors. Citrus zest is perfect for marinades, dressings, and baked goods, adding a burst of freshness to every bite.

iii. **Vinegar**: Vinegar adds acidity and depth to dishes, balancing flavors and cutting through richness. Try different types of vinegar like balsamic, apple cider, or rice vinegar to elevate salads, sauces, and marinades.

iv. **Homemade Sauces and Dressings**: Making your own sauces and dressings allows you to control the ingredients and avoid hidden sugars and unhealthy fats found in store-bought versions. Whip up simple vinaigrettes, creamy yogurt sauces, or tangy salsa fresca to enhance your meals.

- **Cooking Techniques for Blood Sugar Control**

i. **Fiber-Rich Ingredients:** Incorporate plenty of fiber-rich foods like whole grains, legumes, fruits, and vegetables into your recipes. Fiber helps slow down the absorption of sugars into the bloodstream, promoting stable blood sugar levels.

ii. **Portion Control:** Pay attention to portion sizes to prevent overeating and unnecessary spikes in blood sugar. Use smaller plates, bowls, and utensils to help control portion sizes and avoid mindless eating.

iii. **Balanced Meals:** Aim to create balanced meals that include a combination of protein, healthy fats, fiber, and complex carbohydrates. This helps provide sustained energy and keeps you feeling satisfied longer, reducing cravings and the urge to snack on unhealthy foods.

Conclusion

At Trends Kitchen, we understand the importance of not only eating well but also staying active. Combining a balanced diet with regular exercise is key to managing blood sugar levels and promoting overall health and well-being. Yes, you heard that right, incorporating physical activity into your daily routine will help improve insulin sensitivity. It will also allow your body to better regulate blood sugar levels. Aim for at least 30 minutes of moderate-intensity exercise most days of the week. Activities like brisk walking, cycling, swimming, or even dancing can make a significant difference.

When it comes to diet, focus on consuming whole, nutrient-dense foods that provide sustained energy and support optimal blood sugar control. Include plenty of fresh fruits and vegetables, lean proteins, whole grains, and healthy fats in your meals. Avoid highly processed foods, sugary snacks, and excessive amounts of refined carbohydrates, which can cause blood sugar spikes.

Managing stress is also essential for maintaining balanced blood sugar levels. Chronic stress can lead to elevated cortisol levels, which will in turn disrupt insulin production and glucose metabolism. Incorporating stress-reducing practices such as mindfulness meditation, deep breathing exercises, yoga, or spending time in nature helps lower stress levels and improves blood sugar regulation.

Adopting a blood sugar-friendly diet isn't just about managing your immediate health concerns—it's about investing in your long-term well-being. You can reduce your risk of developing chronic conditions such as type 2 diabetes, heart disease, and obesity by making healthier food choices and prioritizing blood sugar control. A balanced diet rich in whole foods also supports weight management, improve energy levels, and enhances overall quality of life.

As you go about controlling your blood sugar better, always have this in mind: small changes lead to significant results over time. Celebrate your progress and don't be too hard on yourself if you slip up occasionally. Every meal is an opportunity to nourish your body and support your health goals.

You will achieve lasting improvements in your blood sugar levels and overall health by staying consistent with your healthy eating habits and incorporating regular physical activity and stress management techniques into your lifestyle. Take control of your health today and enjoy the benefits of a balanced, blood sugar-friendly lifestyle for years to come.

About Trends Kitchen

Trends Kitchen is your go-to source for delicious and nutritious recipes that are as easy to make as they are enjoyable to eat. With a passion for bringing people together through food, Trends Kitchen has dedicated their time to creating accessible and approachable recipes that anyone can enjoy.

The team of seasoned chefs at Trends Kitchen understands the importance of using fresh, high-quality ingredients to create dishes that are both flavorful and nutritious. Their innovative approach to cooking combines traditional flavors with modern techniques, resulting in dishes that are as delicious as they are healthy. In addition to being a culinary haven, Trends Kitchen creates cookbooks, with a number of highly acclaimed titles to their name. Their latest cookbook, the "**Blood Sugar Solution Recipes,**" is proof of their expertise in creating meals that are both delicious and healthy

With a focus on simplicity and accessibility, Trends Kitchen's recipes are designed to inspire home cooks of all skill levels to get creative in the kitchen. Whether you're cooking for yourself or for a crowd, you can trust Trends Kitchen to provide you with the tools and inspiration you need to create meals that are sure to impress. So why wait? Be part of the thousands of satisfied readers who have already discovered the joy of cooking with Trends Kitchen. With their expert guidance and mouthwatering recipes, you'll be on your way to culinary success in no time.

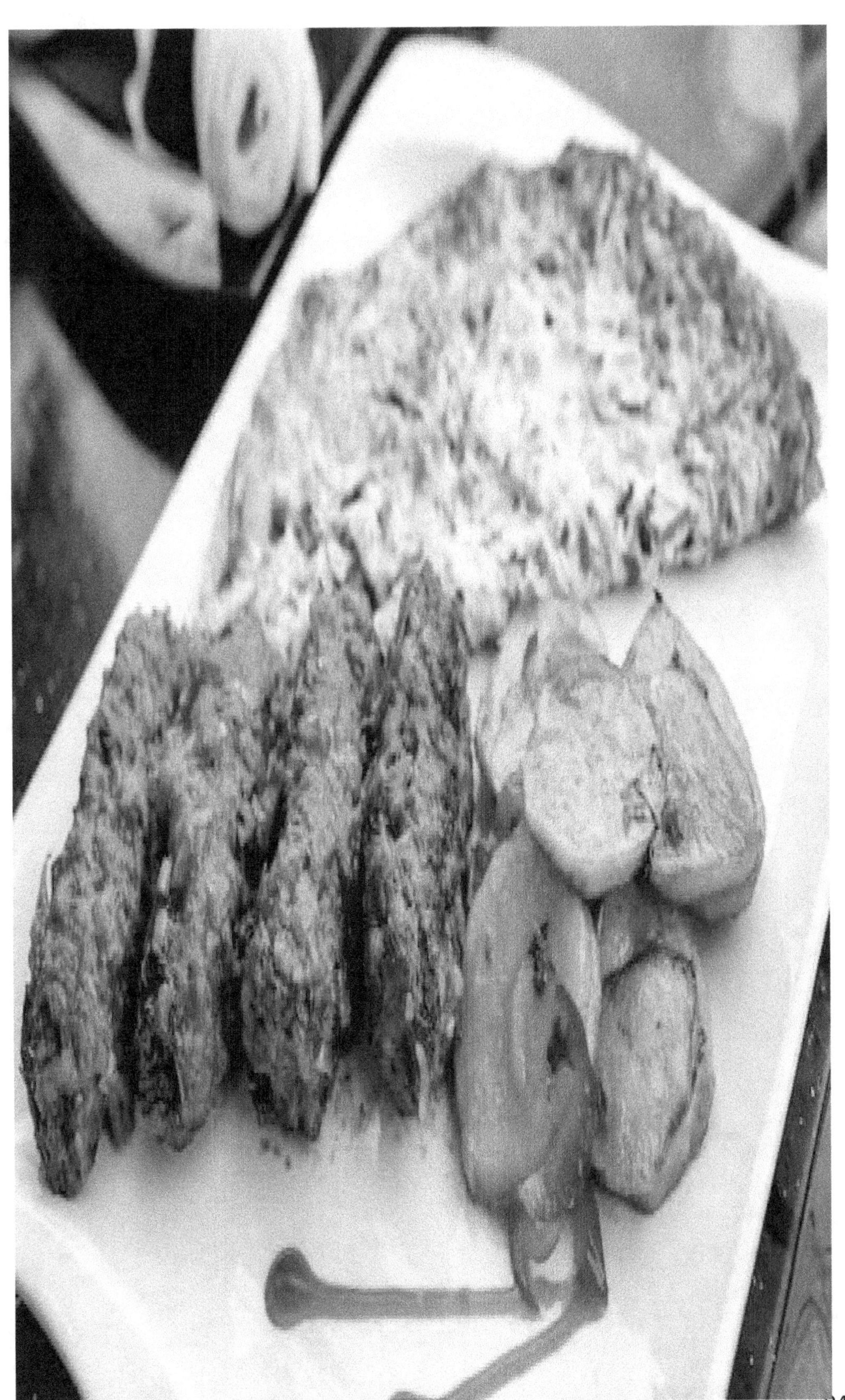

www.ingramcontent.com/pod-product-compliance
Lightning Source LLC
Chambersburg PA
CBHW081223260726
48653CB00010BB/3772